Your Children's Teeth:
A Parent's Guide
To Saving
Money
At The Dentist

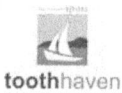

Your Children's Teeth: A Parent's Guide To Saving Money At The Dentist

[2]

Contact Dr. Brazis at (916) 731-5151
Sign Up for To Tell The Tooth Newsletter at:
totellthetooth.com/sign-up

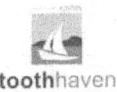

toothhaven

Your Children's Teeth: A Parent's Guide To Saving Money At The Dentist

TABLE OF CONTENTS

Contact Dr. Brazis at (916) 731-5151
Sign Up for To Tell The Tooth Newsletter at:
totellthetooth.com/sign-up

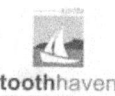

toothhaven

Contact Dr. Brazis at (916) 731-5151
Sign Up for To Tell The Tooth Newsletter at:
totellthetooth.com/sign-up

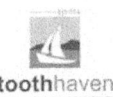

toothhaven

Your Children's Teeth: A Parent's Guide To Saving Money At The Dentist

Contact Dr. Brazis at (916) 731-5151
Sign Up for To Tell The Tooth Newsletter at:
totellthetooth.com/sign-up

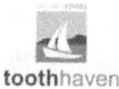

Part-I: Forward

Contact Dr. Brazis at (916) 731-5151
Sign Up for To Tell The Tooth Newsletter at:
totellthetooth.com/sign-up

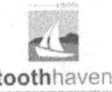

1. About the Author

Dr. Steven J. Brazis attended dental school at the University of the Pacific School of Dentistry in San Francisco and graduated in 1973. He has been practicing general dentistry for over 30 years. He bought his current practice in 1995 and has had a very successful and fulfilling 12 years with mostly the same staff.

Dr. Brazis is a member of the American Dental Association, the California Dental Association and the Sacramento District Dental Society. He is a past member of the San Francisco Dental Society where he also served a term on the Curriculum committee, responsible for the continuing education programs for the society.

Dr. Brazis practices all phases of general dentistry and has had extensive experience in some aspects of oral surgery, but mostly he enjoys having a sense of fulfillment in helping a patient achieve his or her dental goal while

Contact Dr. Brazis at (916) 731-5151
Sign Up for To Tell The Tooth Newsletter at:
totellthetooth.com/sign-up

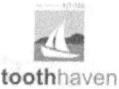
employing the latest technology available to the dental field.

He is married with five grown children and two grandsons . His interests are mostly outdoor sports. He loves backpacking and getting up into the high country of the Sierra Nevada Mountains. He has climbed almost all of the peaks in the Sierra Nevada range between Mt. Whitney and Yosemite at one time. He is an amateur photographer and enjoys computer and internet technology.

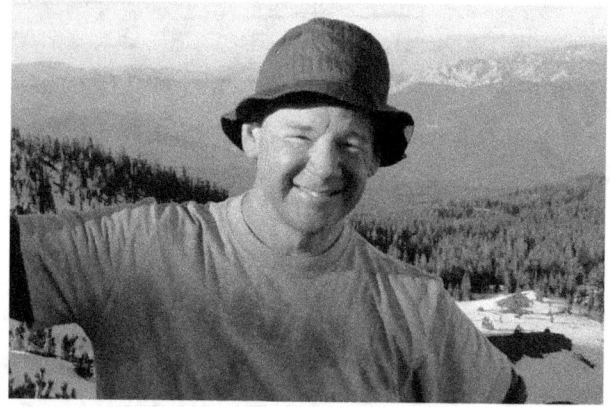

2. Disclaimer

Contact Dr. Brazis at (916) 731-5151
Sign Up for To Tell The Tooth Newsletter at:
totellthetooth.com/sign-up

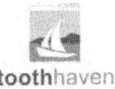
So, this is the part where I tell you what this book is **not**. This book is NOT giving you specific medical or dental advice. It is NOT meant as a second opinion to any advice given by another dentist. Reading this book is NOT an exam with a dentist nor meant to replace one. Your children should be examined regularly by a licensed dentist. You should consult with your dentist if you have any specific questions about your child's dental health. Although, I am a licensed dentist, the information in this book is meant to be for your general knowledge and education so you can better understand your children's dental needs and converse more knowledgeably with your dentist.

Whew!! I hate that part, but there it is. Anyway.....

Contact Dr. Brazis at (916) 731-5151
Sign Up for To Tell The Tooth Newsletter at:
totellthetooth.com/sign-up

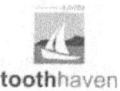

Part-II: Introduction

Contact Dr. Brazis at (916) 731-5151
Sign Up for To Tell The Tooth Newsletter at:
totellthetooth.com/sign-up

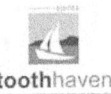

3. Two Stories

In my experience as a dentist, I have met many fine people and their children. I love my job because I get to talk to these people all day long. Most of my patients have met most of my family and are good friends of mine. My wife and one of my daughters have both worked in my office at one time or another.

I have watched children grow up in my practice and then bring their children in to me. However, when I was still young in my practice I had two experiences that I want to share with you. The stories of these two children, though very simple and not at all dramatic, impressed me greatly at the time and I never forgot them.

The publishing of this book is the realization for me of a desire to share information with new parents about their children's dental needs that began with these two very brief encounters and I think you will see why:

[11]

Contact Dr. Brazis at (916) 731-5151
Sign Up for To Tell The Tooth Newsletter at:
totellthetooth.com/sign-up

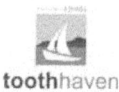

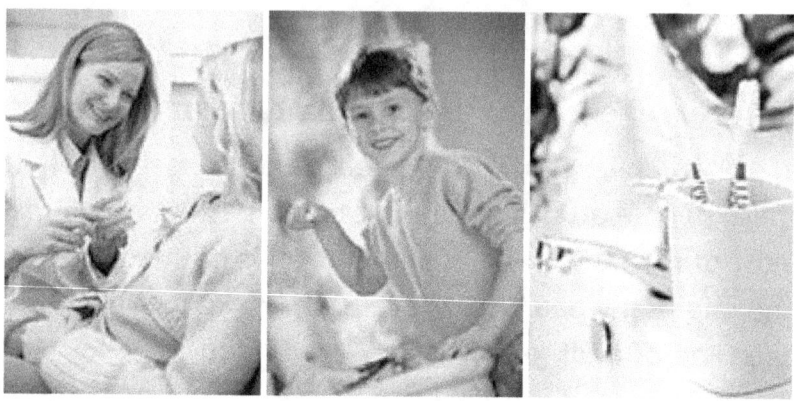

Tommy

Early in my practice of dentistry, a mother brought her young son Tommy to me. Tommy was only 4 1/2 years old, but had massive decay in almost every baby tooth. He was also very shy and very fearful. I told his mother that I would work with him if he let me, but I would not force him to submit to the dental work required. Tommy's mother would not take him to a children's dentist or other specialist, saying she didn't have the money.

[12]

Contact Dr. Brazis at (916) 731-5151
Sign Up for To Tell The Tooth Newsletter at:
totellthetooth.com/sign-up

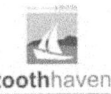

It took me three visits to get Tommy to actually let me finally examine his teeth. He was finally getting to know me and trust me just a little. It was difficult going.

Finally the day came when I was to fix some of his cavities. I was nervous myself at the prospect of causing him any pain and losing the trust we had worked so hard to build in one another. I carefully explained what I was going to do that day, trying to make sure I had eye contact with Tommy to see how he was responding. I noticed that he had his hands jammed in his pockets as I talked and attributed that to nervousness.

As we moved along into the procedure, I came to a point when I needed to get something from my sterilization room while my assistant was helping another patient to get seated. After making sure Tommy was alright to be left alone, I went to get what I needed.

When I returned, I saw Tommy taking his hand away from his mouth. His hand had something dark all over it. I asked

[13]

Contact Dr. Brazis at (916) 731-5151
Sign Up for To Tell The Tooth Newsletter at:
totellthetooth.com/sign-up

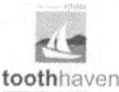
if I could see what he had and he showed me. His hand was covered in chocolate candy! I was shocked. He had been holding the candy in his hand and that was why he had his hands in his pockets. When I left the room, he had put some candy in his mouth.

I went to talk to his mother about this, hoping she didn't even know that Tommy was secretly stuffing candy in his pockets. She told me that she gave it to him because it kept him calm. Besides making me very sad and angry at the same time, that began a deep desire in me to do something to educate parents. Now, many years later, I am blessed with the opportunity to publish this book.

[14]

Contact Dr. Brazis at (916) 731-5151
Sign Up for To Tell The Tooth Newsletter at:
totellthetooth.com/sign-up

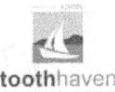
Sarah

This second story is about Doreen and her daughter Sarah. Doreen lived next door to me in San Francisco, CA where I had my practice in those days. She had also become a patient of mine. I had known her when I was a dental student and when I graduated and opened my first practice in downtown San Francisco, it was a natural thing for Doreen to then come to me for her dentistry.

One day Doreen came to the office for a filling. She had brought Sarah with her to the office. After the appointment was finished, it was close to the lunch hour and I had no further appointments for the morning. Doreen asked if she could get my opinion on a neighborhood project she was involved in. I invited her and Sarah into my private office to talk about it.

While Doreen and I were talking, Sarah was playing with some of her toys Doreen had brought with her to keep her busy. After a little bit, Sarah got bored with her toys and began to get a little cranky. After all she had waited

[15]

Contact Dr. Brazis at (916) 731-5151
Sign Up for To Tell The Tooth Newsletter at:
totellthetooth.com/sign-up

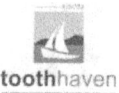
patiently all through her mother's dental appointment after all. Doreen was probably a little cranky herself, from trying to talk and being numb on the right side of her mouth.

Sarah began to play with some dental models of teeth that I had on my desk. Doreen finally turned to Sarah and said something I will never forget. She sharply told Sarah to put those things down and behave herself or "she would have Doctor Steve work on her teeth."

I couldn't believe that Doreen had said that to Sarah, much less right in front of me. I asked her later if she thought that was an appropriate thing to say to her daughter and her response was that Sarah needed to learn to behave herself when in other people's places. It didn't even occur to Doreen that I wasn't talking about reprimanding her daughter, but that I found the reference to dental treatment as a threat of punishment to be inappropriate. To Doreen that was a natural reference. Again, this story points out the need for parent education about the kind of things they say to their children and what impact those

[16]

Contact Dr. Brazis at (916) 731-5151
Sign Up for To Tell The Tooth Newsletter at:
totellthetooth.com/sign-up

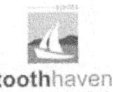
things might have. Admittedly, this was a rather extreme example, but I have heard many parents since then say things about their own dental experience in front of or directly to their children that I know colored that child's impression of dentistry forever.

Children are very impressionable in their early years and the behavior of their parents is what influences them the most. Tommy and Sarah and their mothers were very real people [*though I have changed the names here for privacy of people concerned*]. It is very important to set your children up for success in life in every way possible. Let's look together at how that might be possible where dentistry is concerned and, in the process, save a lot of heartache, pain for your children and money spent at the dentist in the future. (Maybe money isn't everything, but let's face it...it counts.)

===\\\===\\\===\\\===\\\===\\\===\\\===

Contact Dr. Brazis at (916) 731-5151
Sign Up for To Tell The Tooth Newsletter at:
totellthetooth.com/sign-up

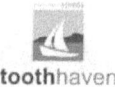
Part-III: Understanding Tooth Development

Contact Dr. Brazis at (916) 731-5151
Sign Up for To Tell The Tooth Newsletter at:
totellthetooth.com/sign-up

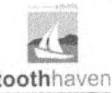

3. Development of Teeth

Development of Primary Teeth

Primary teeth are the first teeth that appear in a baby. These teeth start appearing in your child at around six months of age and often, all primary teeth appear by the time your child is three years old. Whenever I mention ages in this book, remember that these are guidelines only and if your child's teeth are not following this schedule that does not necessarily indicate a problem with their development. If you have any specific questions about their development always ask your dentist.

That said, your baby's teeth start forming in the six-week old fetus. Hard substance in the region where the teeth will appear starts forming at around three to four months of gestation.

Contact Dr. Brazis at (916) 731-5151
Sign Up for To Tell The Tooth Newsletter at:
totellthetooth.com/sign-up

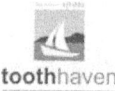
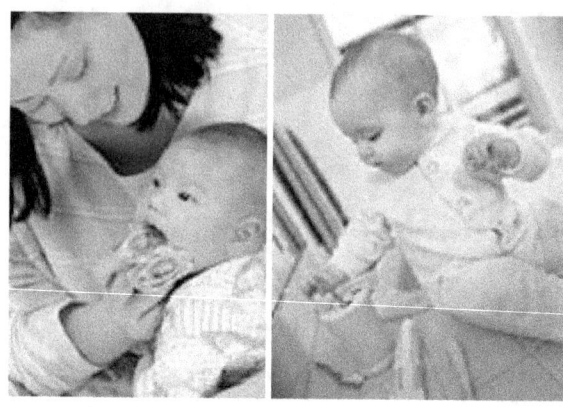

Among the primary teeth, the first to appear are the central incisors (somewhere around six to nine months). These are the front middle teeth. Next, teeth on either side of these central incisors appear, the lateral incisors. Thereafter, the molars appear. Normally, four primary teeth appear every six months. Those in the lower jaw appear ahead of those in the upper jaw. Primary teeth appear in pairs, one on the left side and the other on the right side, though not necessarily at the same time. Girls generally get their primary teeth at an earlier age than boys.

[20]

Contact Dr. Brazis at (916) 731-5151
Sign Up for To Tell The Tooth Newsletter at:
totellthetooth.com/sign-up

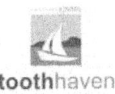
Primary teeth are bright white in color and much smaller than the permanent teeth that appear later. There are only twenty primary teeth in all. Primary teeth form the foundation for the permanent teeth that appear in their place after they fall out. Your child starts the growth and development of the facial and jawbones from the age of four. This could create some spaces in between primary teeth. Spaces help to accommodate the larger permanent teeth, as they appear later. Many parents ask me if these spaces are a problem and indicate the need for braces. The spaces are actually normal and good because it allows the room needed by the larger permanent teeth. There will be enough to worry about later – the spaces are OK!

Although all primary teeth will eventually fall out paving way for permanent teeth, you still want to make sure that you care for these teeth. Healthy teeth are part of your child's overall physical health. They also guide the shape and appearance of facial muscles and structure. These muscles help in efficient chewing and crushing of food. Missing or irregular teeth can disrupt normal chewing of

[21]

Contact Dr. Brazis at (916) 731-5151
Sign Up for To Tell The Tooth Newsletter at:
totellthetooth.com/sign-up

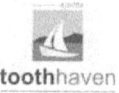

food and lead to food settling between teeth. This could cause tooth decay and gum problems as well as more serious nutritional deficiencies. I can't stress the importance of the baby teeth enough and will return to this later on.

Healthy primary teeth make way for healthy permanent teeth. Tooth infections and decay in primary teeth, although not directly related to problems in the underlying permanent teeth, is a sign of hygiene habits that need to be changed before the arrival of the permanent teeth.

Contact Dr. Brazis at (916) 731-5151
Sign Up for To Tell The Tooth Newsletter at:
totellthetooth.com/sign-up

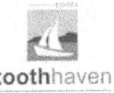

toothhaven

Your Children's Teeth: A Parent's Guide To Saving Money At The Dentist

Eruption (month)	Shedding (year)
Central incisor (8-12)	Central incisor (6-7)
Lateral incisor (9-13)	Lateral incisor (7-8)
Canine/cuspid (16-22)	Canine/cuspid (10-12)
First molar (13-19)	First molar (9-11)
Second molar (25-33)	Second molar (10-12)

Upper

Lower

Eruption (month)	Shedding (year)
Second molar (23-31)	Second molar (10-12)
First molar (14-18)	First molar (9-11)
Canine/cuspid (17-23)	Canine/cuspid (9-12)
Lateral incisor (10-16)	Lateral incisor (7-8)
Central incisor (6-10)	Central incisor (6-7)

[23]

Contact Dr. Brazis at (916) 731-5151
Sign Up for To Tell The Tooth Newsletter at:
totellthetooth.com/sign-up

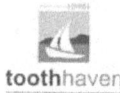
Development of Permanent Teeth

There are 32 permanent teeth in all. These consist of six maxillary (upper) and six mandibular (lower) molars, four maxillary and four mandibular premolars, two maxillary and two mandibular canines, and four maxillary and four mandibular incisors.

In the first set of teeth (primary or baby teeth) there are only 20 teeth (no premolars), whereas there are normally 32 permanent teeth. The three permanent molars (6 year molars, 12 year molars and wisdom teeth) don't replace any baby teeth, but instead come in behind all the baby teeth. Normally, primary teeth start falling out from the age of six and continue until the age of twelve. Permanent teeth push the primary teeth from underneath. However, in between the ages of six and twelve your child will have both primary and permanent teeth. In most cases, all permanent teeth appear by the eighteenth year. In some cases, they may appear until the age of twenty-one.

[24]

Contact Dr. Brazis at (916) 731-5151
Sign Up for To Tell The Tooth Newsletter at:
totellthetooth.com/sign-up

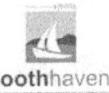
The first primary teeth that start falling are the central incisors (the two front teeth). The first permanent molar could appear by the sixth year. Lateral incisors appear by the eighth year, premolars appear by the ninth and tenth years, while canines appear by the eleventh or twelfth year. The second molar appears by the twelfth or thirteenth year while the third molar appears in between seventeenth and twenty-fifth years (unless they are impacted [stuck] or not present at all).

When primary teeth push out permanent teeth, the jaws and mouth undergo various transformations. These change the shape of your child's face into that of a growing adult. Permanent teeth grow to a certain size. Thereafter, the root closes, and teeth stop growing.

Contact Dr. Brazis at (916) 731-5151
Sign Up for To Tell The Tooth Newsletter at:
totellthetooth.com/sign-up

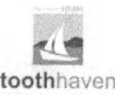
Your Children's Teeth: A Parent's Guide To Saving Money At The Dentist

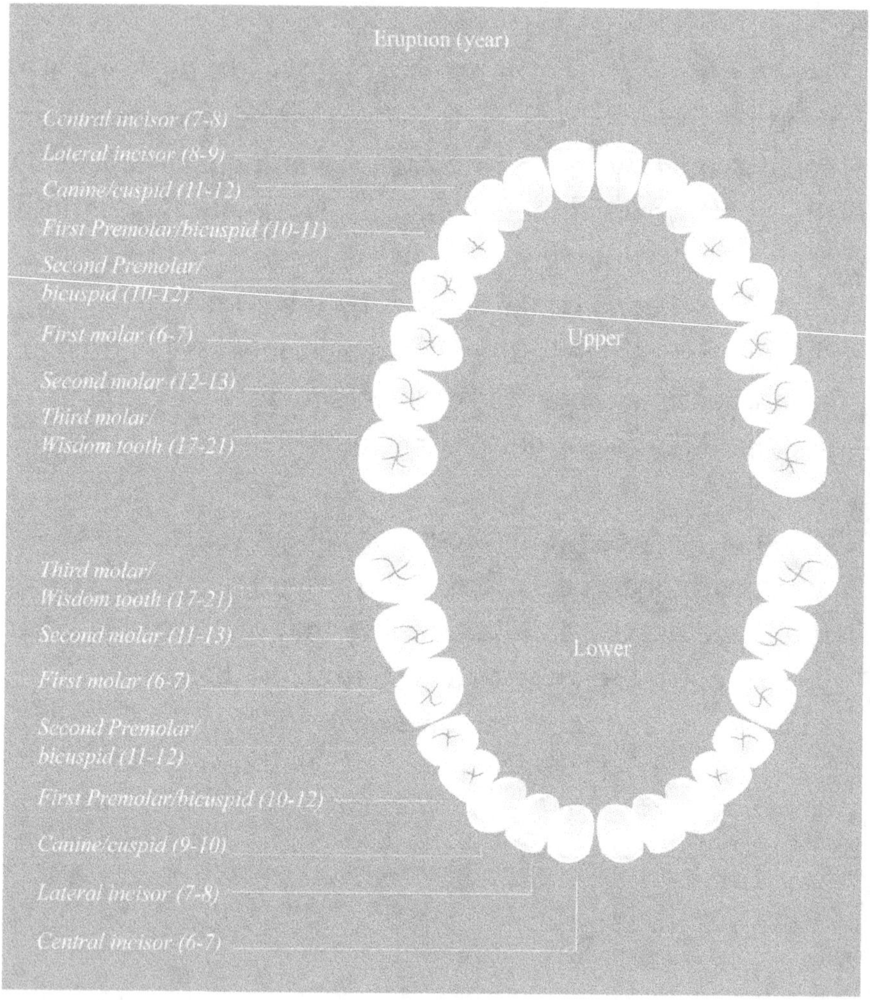

Eruption (year)

Central incisor (7-8)
Lateral incisor (8-9)
Canine/cuspid (11-12)
First Premolar/bicuspid (10-11)
Second Premolar/
bicuspid (10-12)
First molar (6-7)
Second molar (12-13)
Third molar/
Wisdom tooth (17-21)

Upper

Third molar/
Wisdom tooth (17-21)
Second molar (11-13)
First molar (6-7)
Second Premolar/
bicuspid (11-12)
First Premolar/bicuspid (10-12)
Canine/cuspid (9-10)
Lateral incisor (7-8)
Central incisor (6-7)

Lower

[26]

Contact Dr. Brazis at (916) 731-5151
Sign Up for To Tell The Tooth Newsletter at:
totellthetooth.com/sign-up

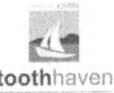

Jaw Development

Although the following discussion is a little more technical than most parents ask about, I am including it here to give you a better idea of your child's physical growth and development.

The bones of the upper and lower jaws form the foundation for growth and development of teeth. They are responsible for overall dental development. The Maxilla is the upper jaw and the Mandible is the lower jaw. These are the strongest and largest bones of the face and hence are the main supporters of teeth.

Both the maxilla and mandible have two different types of bones. The basal bone forms the foundation of dental skeletal structure and alveolar bone provides the hard support necessary for supporting teeth. Good quality of the alveolar bone protects your teeth from diseases and any other trauma.

[27]

Contact Dr. Brazis at (916) 731-5151
Sign Up for To Tell The Tooth Newsletter at:
totellthetooth.com/sign-up

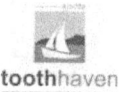

The maxilla consists of two bones. It acts as a fitter for accommodating all other facial bones. It holds the floor and lateral nose wall, roof of mouth, and bony eye cavity with all muscles, nerves, and blood vessels. There are four parts of each bone with four surfaces: posterior (back), anterior (front), lateral (outer), and medial (inner).

Mandible is the bone structure of the lower jaw. It is the only bone of human skull and face, which moves. It accommodates the lower set of teeth in your mouth. It has a curved horizontal shape, similar to a horseshoe. The mandible jaw has two surfaces, internal and external and two borders, superior and inferior. The mandible forms a bilateral (both sides of the body) joint with the temporal bones of the skull with a soft cartilaginous disc between the ball of the mandible and the fossa (socket) of the temporal bones.

Contact Dr. Brazis at (916) 731-5151
Sign Up for To Tell The Tooth Newsletter at:
totellthetooth.com/sign-up

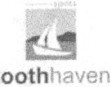
===\\\===\\\===\\\===\\\===\\\===\\\===

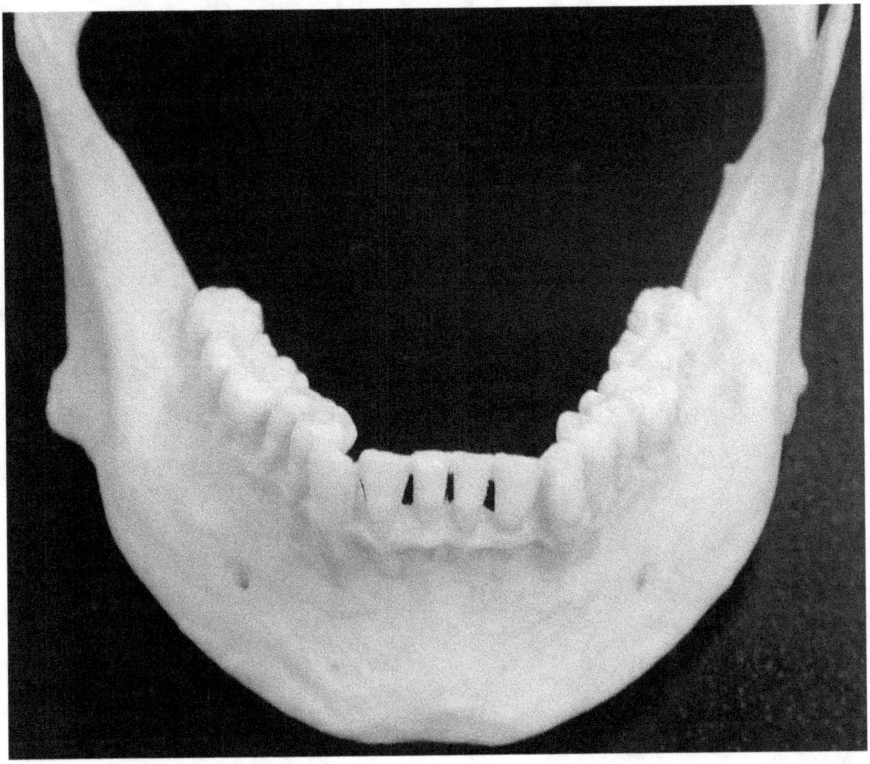

[29]

Contact Dr. Brazis at (916) 731-5151
Sign Up for To Tell The Tooth Newsletter at:
totellthetooth.com/sign-up

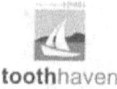
4. How to Help Your Child When Teething

Teeth start appearing in your infant from six months of age approximately. But they will start feeling them a few months before this. Children prefer gnawing at any hard objects during teething. It could also cause excessive drooling.

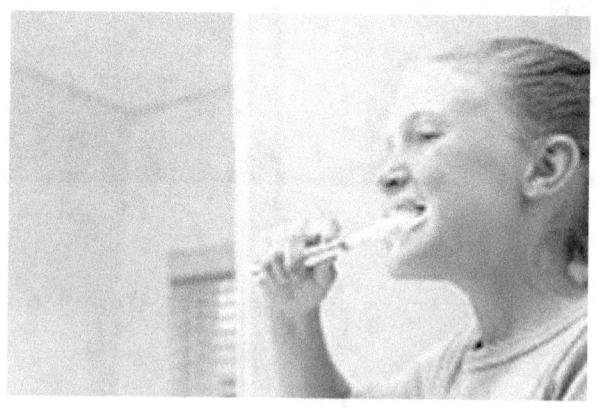

[30]

Contact Dr. Brazis at (916) 731-5151
Sign Up for To Tell The Tooth Newsletter at:
totellthetooth.com/sign-up

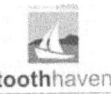
toothhaven

Teething is a very uncomfortable and painful experience for most infants and toddlers. Gums could become tender and swollen. Often your baby's cheeks turn deep red near the gums. Your child could become cranky and irritable and wake up crying at night (this is fun for the whole family). Some of these symptoms can also be signs of other problems besides teething. It never hurts to call your doctor if you have any questions. Although you cannot prevent teething problems, you can provide some relief.

Some Simple Helpful Tactics

- You can give your child a chilled teething ring to ease pain and irritation, but do <u>not</u> give them frozen teething rings. This could cause frostbites to gums and lips.

- You can use a cold spoon or clean wet finger to rub your child's gums gently.

- Wrap some ice in a clean washcloth and allow your child to chew it.

[31]

Contact Dr. Brazis at (916) 731-5151
Sign Up for To Tell The Tooth Newsletter at:
totellthetooth.com/sign-up

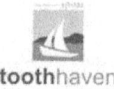
toothhaven

Your Children's Teeth: A Parent's Guide To Saving Money At The Dentist

- Offer them a cold celery stick or cold carrot for chewing. However, keep a close eye on your child to prevent any choking due to soft carrot pieces.

- You don't want to give them hard foods like frozen bananas. This can cause gum abrasions or laceration.

- Diarrhea, vomiting, high fever, and irregular sleeping patterns can be but are not necessarily associated with teething. These symptoms could be for different ailments altogether. Don't hesitate to check with your pediatrician. This is an important time in your baby's life and they can't tell you yet what is bothering them (though they try like heck).

===\\\===\\\===\\\===\\\===\\\===\\\===

[32]

Contact Dr. Brazis at (916) 731-5151
Sign Up for To Tell The Tooth Newsletter at:
totellthetooth.com/sign-up

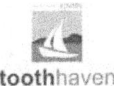

Your Children's Teeth: A Parent's Guide To Saving Money At The Dentist

Part-IV: Dental Care at Home

Contact Dr. Brazis at (916) 731-5151
Sign Up for To Tell The Tooth Newsletter at:
totellthetooth.com/sign-up

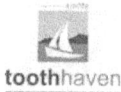
5. Cleaning Your Child's Mouth and Teeth

Importance of Baby Teeth

Baby teeth or primary teeth are of paramount importance. Primary teeth are often inadequately cared for in the belief that they will fall out and permanent teeth will come in their place. *Remember little Tommy.* If you do not take care of these primary teeth, they may end up having to be extracted. This could cause irregular alignment and/or crowding of the permanent teeth coming in their place. This might cause problems later in life (which can lead to hefty orthodontic bills.) Lack of care may also lead to abscess formation, which can affect the bone support for the permanent teeth later on. Painful and missing baby teeth can also cause severe nutritional problems. *(Told you we'd get back to this - Baby Teeth are <u>IMPORTANT</u>!!)*

Contact Dr. Brazis at (916) 731-5151
Sign Up for To Tell The Tooth Newsletter at:
totellthetooth.com/sign-up

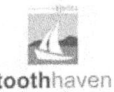

toothhaven

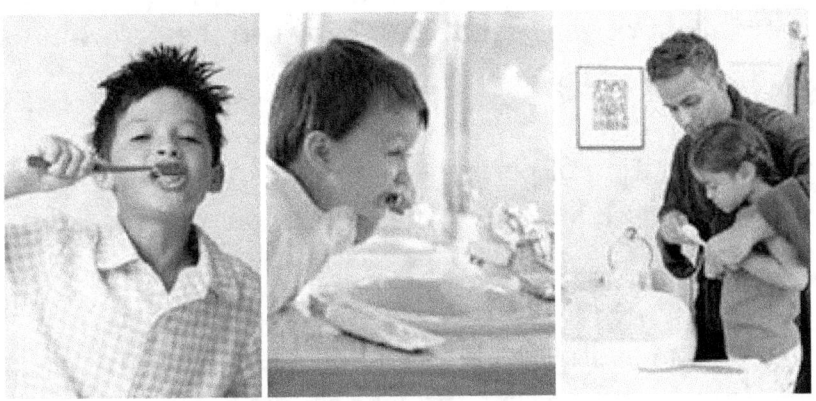

Parents often ask me about the spacing of their children's baby teeth and the need for orthodontics. Baby teeth often grow at spaced intervals with spaces between them. This allows your child to grow permanent teeth in an even and phased manner. This promotes natural formation of facial muscles and jawbones. A good indication for whether orthodontics will be appropriate is the position of the first permanent molars. This is something your dentist can asses and advise you on.

A good set of teeth helps your child eat all types of food. This provides essential nutrition for overall growth and

[35]

Contact Dr. Brazis at (916) 731-5151
Sign Up for To Tell The Tooth Newsletter at:
totellthetooth.com/sign-up

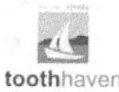
development of your child. Your baby can then grow into a healthy child and a healthy individual.

Proper formation of permanent teeth is essential to give shape to your child's face. They make your child look attractive and beautiful. Baby teeth lay the foundation for a lifetime of beautiful teeth, good dental hygiene, healthy jaws, and an overall good-looking face and healthy individual. Hence, caring for your child's baby teeth is essential and starts right from the womb.

Early Care of Your Child's Teeth

Teeth start forming in the second trimester of pregnancy. This might be a good time to mention a few things about pregnancy. As a soon to be mother, you are eating for two. You should be making sure to get the proper amounts of vitamins A, C, D and Phosphorus and Calcium either through diet or supplementation. Eating fruits, leafy vegetables and low-fat dairy products will help. Get plenty of protein in your diet.

[36]

Contact Dr. Brazis at (916) 731-5151
Sign Up for To Tell The Tooth Newsletter at:
totellthetooth.com/sign-up

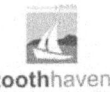
The increase in progesterone hormone causes you to become more prone to gum irritation and disease at this time. You should be especially diligent with your own home care (brushing, flossing and drinking plenty of water). Gum disease has been linked to diabetic complications, stroke and heart disease. It has also been linked to premature delivery, which can be a serious problem for your baby.

At birth, your baby has twenty primary teeth, which remain well developed within the jaw, though not yet visible in the mouth. Caring for your child's teeth should start very early, even before there are any signs of tooth formation and eruption.

Avoid bottle feeding your child while they sleep. Use a soft wet-cloth or gauze pad wound around your finger to wipe your infant's gums after every feeding. You can also use a terrycloth finger-cot available at most drugstores for wiping gums. This removes any leftover food and keeps gums clean and free of bacterial deposits. Use a very soft

[37]

Contact Dr. Brazis at (916) 731-5151
Sign Up for To Tell The Tooth Newsletter at:
totellthetooth.com/sign-up

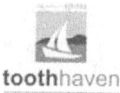
toothbrush to brush your child's teeth once small baby teeth start coming out.

Once small primary teeth start appearing, be sure to clean along gum-line. This is where most plaque deposits start. Plaque deposits lead to cavities, tooth decay, and inflamed gums.

Initially, brush with water only. Thereafter, use very little toothpaste on brush. Continue brushing your baby's teeth like this morning and evening until your child is around three years old. Again, this is a guideline only. Some kids mature a little faster, some take a little longer. My oldest grandson was playing with his toothbrush at two. He's always wanted to do everything himself rather than have anything done for him, bless his little heart.

You will want to start flossing your child's teeth when they are in tight contact. Flossing cleans in between teeth. Toothbrush bristles cannot reach here. Any deposits here

Contact Dr. Brazis at (916) 731-5151
Sign Up for To Tell The Tooth Newsletter at:
totellthetooth.com/sign-up

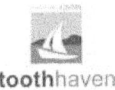
can lead to tooth cavities and later decay. Teach your child the correct flossing techniques.

Until the age of three, you should brush your child's teeth morning and night. Thereafter, you can start teaching brushing and essential dental habits to your child. Your child may brush teeth once and you can do the other time. This ensures thorough cleaning of your child's teeth and at the same time, you can teach your child to brush teeth independently.

Toothbrushes should be according to your child's age. Brushing with a small head helps in complete cleaning all through the gum line. Brushes with soft bristles are the best as they do not damage or harm gums.

How to Get Your Child to Brush

Brushing teeth twice everyday should become a regular habit in your child. This prevents most dental problems. I

[39]

Contact Dr. Brazis at (916) 731-5151
Sign Up for To Tell The Tooth Newsletter at:
totellthetooth.com/sign-up

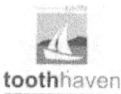
offer here some suggestions to make this an easy and fun accomplishment for your child:

- As a concerned parent, start good oral habits in your child soon after birth. Regular cleaning and wiping of your child's mouth after every feed gets your baby used to you to cleaning his/her mouth. This also makes it easier for a dentist to examine your child's mouth later on.

- You should brush your child's teeth in the initial years. Regular brushing makes your child accustomed to a clean mouth. Your child soon understands and appreciates a clean mouth. They also appreciate snacks and treats, so the sooner the habits are begun, the more likely they will be to follow through later. Brushing then becomes a regular habit, hopefully even after the snacks and treats.

- As your child grows, use very little toothpaste on a soft brush to teach proper brushing of teeth. Putting a small amount of toothpaste restricts foam formation and makes it easier for your child to brush teeth.

Contact Dr. Brazis at (916) 731-5151
Sign Up for To Tell The Tooth Newsletter at:
totellthetooth.com/sign-up

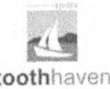

toothhaven

Your Children's Teeth: A Parent's Guide To Saving Money At The Dentist

- As they get a little older allow them to brush their own teeth and you can either finish up for them or allow them to brush their teeth in the mornings and you can brush their teeth at night.

- Make brushing a fun affair by including elder siblings. Otherwise, parents can brush teeth together making lot of noise and indulge in few teeth brushing games. Children will join in the fun and start enjoying their tooth brushing sessions. Practice good dental habits in the family. Children love to copy their elders. This will help them develop their own good dental habits.

===\\\===\\\===\\\===\\\===\\\===\\\===

[41]

Contact Dr. Brazis at (916) 731-5151
Sign Up for To Tell The Tooth Newsletter at:
totellthetooth.com/sign-up

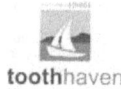
6. How to Care for Your Child's Teeth

Fluoride has been shown to have definite beneficial effects on the growth of strong teeth, as it hardens tooth enamel. Fluoride in higher doses has also been shown to be detrimental to health in other ways. The controversy over fluoride rages on today. You will have to make your own decisions about the use of supplemental fluoride, as there are compelling arguments on both sides of the controversy. For more on this go to:

http://www.toothhaven.com/?p=38.

Normally, tap water in most cities contains some fluoride supplementation. Otherwise, you could ask your doctor to prescribe fluoride tablets for regular and daily use. However, to avoid possibility of harmful effects do not

[42]

Contact Dr. Brazis at (916) 731-5151
Sign Up for To Tell The Tooth Newsletter at:
totellthetooth.com/sign-up

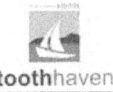
exceed recommended doses of fluoride. Never use Fluoride supplements without the recommendation and guidance of a pediatrician or pedodontist.

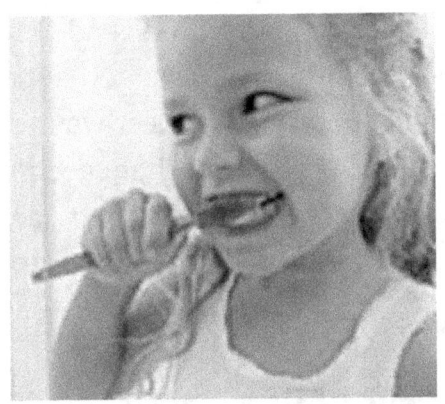

Cavities are the most common dental problem among children. If you allow your infant to sleep with a bottle of milk or juice, sugar present in milk or juice can remain on the gums and teeth for a prolonged period. This leads to cavities. Don't allow your child to walk around all waking hours with a bottle. Instead, teach your child to start drinking from a cup as soon as they are able.

[43]

Contact Dr. Brazis at (916) 731-5151
Sign Up for To Tell The Tooth Newsletter at:
totellthetooth.com/sign-up

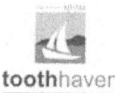
Additionally, if your child consumes lots of sugary foods like candy, cookies, raisins, and many sweetened fruit juices, there is a high risk of developing cavities. If most of your family members suffer from cavities, your child could also develop cavities early in life. The tendency towards tooth decay may be hereditary, but the actual development of cavities requires bacteria. The best way to take good care of your child's teeth is to feed them good nutritious non-sweetened foods and brush regularly twice every day, in the morning and at bedtime. Flossing once a day is equally essential.

Caring for Your Child's Teeth – Before Birth to 6 Months

- A healthy pregnancy contributes to healthy formation of teeth in your baby. A woman should eat a nutritious and balanced diet with lots of vitamins and minerals during her pregnancy. She should also, undergo a thorough dental examination and have any decayed teeth filled or oral infections resolved. Your baby's teeth start forming from

[44]

Contact Dr. Brazis at (916) 731-5151
Sign Up for To Tell The Tooth Newsletter at:
totellthetooth.com/sign-up

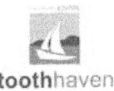
the second trimester of-pregnancy. A baby at birth has all twenty teeth, although within the jaws beneath the gums.

- After the birth of your child, in addition to a good nutritious diet, follow simple dental habits. As I said earlier if you are bottle-feeding your child, do not let them sleep with the bottle. Sugars from juice and milk stay for prolonged periods and cause bacteria to develop. Remove bottle soon after feeding.

- Clean your child's mouth and gums with a wet gauze after feedings and at bedtime. If anyone in the household smokes, you will want to keep your child away from the tobacco and cigarette smoke. Aside from the obvious harmful medical effects, this could cause gum inflammation.

Caring for Your Child's Teeth - 6 Months to 3 Years

[45]

Contact Dr. Brazis at (916) 731-5151
Sign Up for To Tell The Tooth Newsletter at:
totellthetooth.com/sign-up

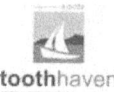

- Infants start the eruption of their first teeth from the age of six months. They normally have six teeth around their first birthday. Use a wet cloth or sponge to wipe their gums after feedings. After the first few teeth appear, use a soft brush and water to clean your infant's teeth. Develop the habit of drinking from a cup around nine months of age to discourage bottle-feeds.

- Put a pea-sized amount of toothpaste on the toothbrush to brush your child's teeth after your child is a year-old. Until the age of three, you should brush your child's teeth both in the morning and at night. Teach your child not to swallow toothpaste.

- Develop good eating habits in your child by giving foods that help in growth and development of strong gums and teeth like fruits, vegetables, and whole grains. Avoid sugary or high-carbohydrate foods like pastries, pasta, and processed carbohydrates.

[46]

Contact Dr. Brazis at (916) 731-5151
Sign Up for To Tell The Tooth Newsletter at:
totellthetooth.com/sign-up

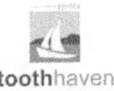
Caring for Your Child's Teeth - 3 Years to 6 Years

- At three years of age, your child may be learning to talk and starting to understand a few things. This is a good time to teach your child good dental habits.

  One day my own grandson, Christian and I were talking. He calls me Peepaw. He said, " Peepaw, my mom doesn't want me to eat at McDonalds. How come?" Wow! So I told him some things about good and bad foods and why they were good or bad. I was amazed that he was listening. (How come my kids didn't when they were his age...oh, well. That's another discussion.) Anyway, he then said that he was going to only eat good foods like vegetables. I wish, but he was listening (and I hope, remembering).

- Teach your child to brush their teeth on their own with your supervision. You can encourage your child to watch

[47]

Contact Dr. Brazis at (916) 731-5151
Sign Up for To Tell The Tooth Newsletter at:
totellthetooth.com/sign-up

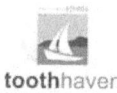
other elder siblings and elders brushing their teeth to learn the correct techniques.

- Flossing is essential as soon as teeth start touching each other. Use plastic flossing tools available in the market to teach proper flossing habits to your child.

- Infants and small children often suck their thumbs. A four-year old normally stops thumb sucking on their own. If not, you can take necessary guidance from your dentist to stop this habit and avoid unnecessary orthodontic complications.

- These discussions and habits at this early age can end up saving hundreds (or thousands) of dollars in dental visits later on.

Caring for Your Child's Teeth - 6 Years to 16 Years

- From the age of six, your child starts losing all primary teeth and permanent teeth start growing in their place. By

[48]

Contact Dr. Brazis at (916) 731-5151
Sign Up for To Tell The Tooth Newsletter at:
totellthetooth.com/sign-up

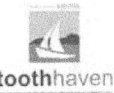

now, your child should be able to brush their own teeth independently. Help your child realize the importance of brushing regularly in the morning and evening. They may not act like it, but they are listening. Teach your child to floss regularly. <u>You can ask your dentist to guide your child</u> on correct technique of flossing.

- Take your child to the dentist regularly. If your child develops cavities, the dentist will suggest proper treatment remedies. Give chewable disclosing tablets to your child regularly to detect any plaque left on your child's teeth after brushing. These are available at local drugstores. They cause the plaque on the teeth to stain red so that it can be seen. This can also make brushing a fun game, by the way.

- You can discuss with your dentist if it is essential to put dental sealants on the molar teeth of your child. Sealants are of hard plastic. They protect chewing surfaces of your child's teeth from decay.

Contact Dr. Brazis at (916) 731-5151
Sign Up for To Tell The Tooth Newsletter at:
totellthetooth.com/sign-up

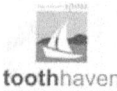

toothhaven

- Teach your child to eat nutritious food like fruits, vegetables, and whole grains. Educate your child about ill effects of highly processed carbohydrates and sugary foods. This paves the way for healthy dental care in your youngster. Yes, it would help if you eat that way as well. I know, I like tasty snacks also. But remember that your kids can only eat what you buy for them, at least until they get older. Hopefully by then the habits will be ingrained.

===\\\===\\\===\\\===\\\===\\\===\\\===

Contact Dr. Brazis at (916) 731-5151
Sign Up for To Tell The Tooth Newsletter at:
totellthetooth.com/sign-up

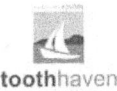

toothhaven

7. Parenting Tips on Use of Pacifiers, Dental Sealants, and Candy Eating

Thumb sucking and pacifiers are very similar habits with very different problems associated with them:

Is Your Child Thumb Sucking or Using a Pacifier?

Thumb sucking or use of pacifier is common among babies and young children. This habit starts from the time your child is in the womb as embryos suck on thumbs. Pacifiers and thumb sucking make children feel secure and comfortable as if sucking on their mother's nipple.

[51]

Contact Dr. Brazis at (916) 731-5151
Sign Up for To Tell The Tooth Newsletter at:
totellthetooth.com/sign-up

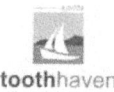
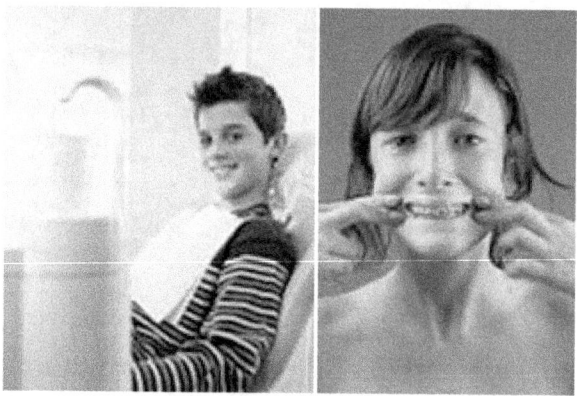

Pacifiers should be solid and molded as a single piece and not as two separate pieces joined. The nipple end of a pacifier should not be brittle. These could lead to choking incidents. Do <u>not</u> tie the pacifier around your child's neck, as it could cause strangulation. Do not encourage any dipped pacifiers for your child, as these often contain honey as a dipper. This also causes tooth decay.

Children normally outgrow their thumb sucking habits before the age of four or five. As permanent teeth start coming only around the age of six, thumb-sucking usually won't cause any problems.

[52]

Contact Dr. Brazis at (916) 731-5151
Sign Up for To Tell The Tooth Newsletter at:
totellthetooth.com/sign-up

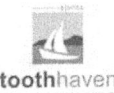

If they have not stopped thumb sucking by the time the permanent central incisors have arrived, ask your dentist for suggestions.

Is Candy the Only Enemy of Your Child's Healthy Teeth?

Candy is the main cause of dental cavities in children. Most parents prefer children eating other healthier snacks. However, the so-called healthier snacks are not entirely safe either.

Cavities occur due to food residue on teeth. Bacteria act upon such food materials and produce an acid. This acid eats into tooth enamel and causes decay. Hence, to avoid cavities, you should keep your child's teeth clean and free of all food residues.

All snacks like potato chips, raisins, pasta, peanut butter, and fruits contain a lot of carbohydrates. Along with

[53]

Contact Dr. Brazis at (916) 731-5151
Sign Up for To Tell The Tooth Newsletter at:
totellthetooth.com/sign-up

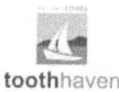
sugars, they are equally responsible for creating cavities. As they stick to teeth, they provide the necessary residue for bacterial plaque formation.

Although candy and other similar food are equally responsible for causing dental cavities, candy is considered more harmful. This is because although candy provides energy, it <u>does not provide any other essential nutrients</u>. Hence, regular candy consumption will deprive your child's body of other essential nutrients like proteins, fats, and minerals. All these are necessary for overall development.

Restrict eating of candy in your children. Right, not easy but, remember, you're doing it for them (and your pocket book.) Allow them to have candy only if they have eaten nutritious well-balanced meals, and even then, not on a regular basis. Provide healthier snacks like yogurt and nuts. However, make sure your kids understand the importance of brushing teeth after every meal and after snacks as well. This can save them from dental cavities and other problems.

[54]

Contact Dr. Brazis at (916) 731-5151
Sign Up for To Tell The Tooth Newsletter at:
totellthetooth.com/sign-up

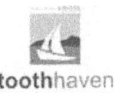

Dental Sealants and Childhood Cavities

Sealants were mentioned earlier but they are of such great value as a preventive measure that I want to take a minute to discuss their benefits further. The vast majority of cavities that people suffer from began in their childhood years between the ages of 4 and 18. Use of fluoride toothpastes and supplements has reduced childhood dental cavities largely. Yet, children do still suffer from dental cavities (caries). Dentists recommend use of dental sealants to overcome this problem.

Cavities are predominant in molar teeth present at the back of the mouth. These molars have small grooves and pits that accumulate food deposits and bacterial plaque. These plaque deposits are difficult if not impossible to remove with traditional brushing or flossing because of the extremely small size of these fissures and pits. This acids produced by this *hidden* plaque acts on tooth enamel and causes dental cavities.

[55]

Contact Dr. Brazis at (916) 731-5151
Sign Up for To Tell The Tooth Newsletter at:
totellthetooth.com/sign-up

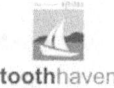
Dentists clean molar tooth surfaces thoroughly and prepare them for application of dental sealants. These sealants are nontoxic and clear or tooth colored. Dentists flow this sealant into these pits and fissures. This disallows any food material to settle in and invite bacteria.

Application process of dental sealants is simple and painless. Once applied, sealants remain in place for four to five years. Thereafter, dentists reapply them effortlessly. Normally dentists recommend application of dental sealants once your child is over six years.

American Dental Association supports application and use of dental sealants in children. These are very effective against dental cavities. Yet, the percentage of children receiving dental sealants is very low. This is mainly due to lack of awareness regarding benefits of dental sealants.

===\\\===\\\===\\\===\\\===\\\===\\\===

[56]

Contact Dr. Brazis at (916) 731-5151
Sign Up for To Tell The Tooth Newsletter at:
totellthetooth.com/sign-up

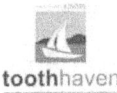

8. Nutrition and Dental Health - Feeding Your Child Tooth-Friendly Foods

In this day and age of fast and processed foods it can be a challenge to ensure a healthy diet for your family. Everyone wants to provide good food for their families, but how to do that when the stores are full of processed foods and fast food chains are everywhere boggles the mind. However, for the parent willing to look, there are good whole food and health food stores also. Look for foods that are high in fiber and nutrients and low in chemical additives and sugars.

Contact Dr. Brazis at (916) 731-5151
Sign Up for To Tell The Tooth Newsletter at:
totellthetooth.com/sign-up

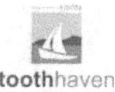

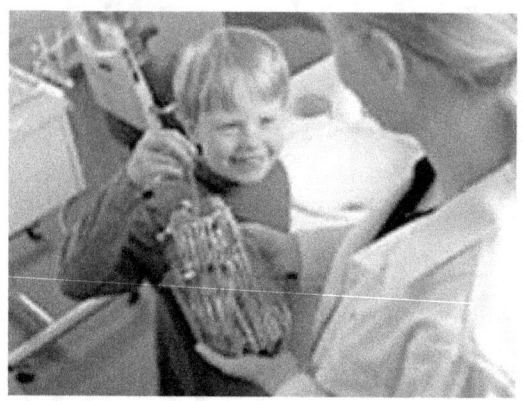

Some suggestions for finding excellent health foods and snacks online:

- http://www.sunfood.com

Essential Nutritious Food

Children are in their growing stages and therefore require foods from each food group to maintain proper health. Include carbohydrates, proteins, and fats in every meal. Normally, a child's diet has a higher concentration of

[58]

Contact Dr. Brazis at (916) 731-5151
Sign Up for To Tell The Tooth Newsletter at:
totellthetooth.com/sign-up

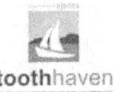

carbohydrates. Carbohydrates contain starches and sugars, some harmful and some essential. Try to emphasize the complex carbohydrates found in vegetables and fruits as opposed to the starchy carbohydrates found in pasta and breads.

All types of foods and snacks are able to cause dental cavities. Cookies, candies, pastries, and cakes are the obvious troublemakers. Yet, fruits, milk, peanut butter, pretzels, chips, and juices are equally detrimental. Regulating eating habits along with regular brushing habits will help tremendously.

Water

Water is a subject that is so often overlooked in discussions of nutrition that I want to give it special attention here. If you give your child water to drink early on in life instead of flavored drinks of any kind, they will grow up to appreciate water and want to drink it naturally. Most people do not get enough good water in their bodies. Water is a natural

Contact Dr. Brazis at (916) 731-5151
Sign Up for To Tell The Tooth Newsletter at:
totellthetooth.com/sign-up

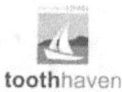
lubricant and cleanser. It is a necessary catalyst for most of the essential metabolism of the body as well as acting as a cleansing agent to flush waste and toxic materials from the cells and body as a whole.

Today, most water sources need extra filtering to make sure it doesn't contain more harmful ingredients than good. Bottled water is an alternative, though that can be expensive. Good inexpensive water filters can be found with a little research and well worth the effort.

Finally, just drinking water during and after eating will wash out the mouth and help dilute any remaining food substance left, reducing the risk of tooth decay enormously.

Tips to Maintain Good Dental Health in Children

[60]

Contact Dr. Brazis at (916) 731-5151
Sign Up for To Tell The Tooth Newsletter at:
totellthetooth.com/sign-up

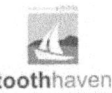

Your Children's Teeth: A Parent's Guide To Saving Money At The Dentist

- Avoid giving sticky food like raisins, honey, caramel, syrups, and molasses to children. Otherwise, insist on your children brushing their teeth immediately after eating such foods.

- Give them raw vegetables and fruits for snacks. Vegetables and fruits like cucumber, pear, celery, and melon stimulate the secretion of saliva during eating. This helps wash away sugars present in such fruits and vegetables and prevent any buildup of food residue.

- Give cheddar cheese as an alternative snack or for lunch. This triggers saliva formation and helps wash down food particles. *Go to the following link for source article*: http://www.toothhaven.com/?p=40.

- Give children water instead of juices or soda. Juices and soda have high levels of sugar. Soda also has carbolic acid, which is extremely destructive to teeth. Diluting fruit juices with some water is also helpful.

[61]

Contact Dr. Brazis at (916) 731-5151
Sign Up for To Tell The Tooth Newsletter at:
totellthetooth.com/sign-up

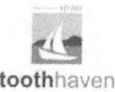

- Use a fluoridated toothpaste if you choose for brushing. Fluoride helps improve the hardness of enamel and prevents tooth decay. Flossing removes food deposits between the teeth where brushing cannot.

- It is best to brush teeth well twice a day and preferably also after meals and snacks. Drink lots of water!

===\\\===\\\===\\\===\\\===\\\===\\\===

Contact Dr. Brazis at (916) 731-5151
Sign Up for To Tell The Tooth Newsletter at:
totellthetooth.com/sign-up

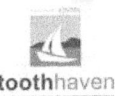
9. Choosing Dental Care Products for Your Child

There are many dental care products: toothpastes, mouthwashes, toothbrushes, mouth rinses teething rings, and pacifiers, etc. You should be careful in choosing products for your children. Consult your dentist about dental care products for your child.

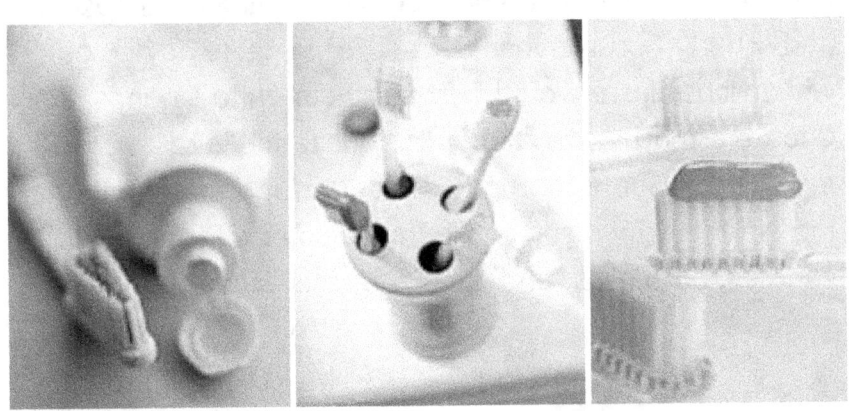

[63]

Contact Dr. Brazis at (916) 731-5151
Sign Up for To Tell The Tooth Newsletter at:
totellthetooth.com/sign-up

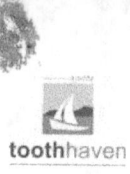

toothhaven

Toothpaste

While purchasing toothpaste, look for product approval seal of American Dental Association. This seal certifies that the toothpaste is safe and effective for all scientifically proven claims. Toothpastes usually have a manufacturer's label proclaiming age suitability for use. Often young children tend to swallow toothpaste. Monitoring their brushing, you can help discourage this.

There are numerous other types of toothpastes like tartar-control, desensitizing, gum care, whitening toothpastes, and others. Consult your dentist for suitable advice on which toothpaste would best suit your child's needs. Choose a toothpaste that suits your family's tastes and needs best. Some toothpastes contain spearmint or other ingredients which can cause irritation or allergy in your child's mouth, lips, and cheeks. If this occurs, switch brands.

Contact Dr. Brazis at (916) 731-5151
Sign Up for To Tell The Tooth Newsletter at:
totellthetooth.com/sign-up

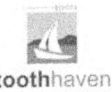

Toothbrush

Toothbrushes should always have soft bristles. Hard bristles harm gums and jaws. The toothbrush head should be able to brush two teeth at a time. Children and infants require toothbrushes with smaller heads so that they fit into their mouths easily and allow thorough cleaning of all teeth. Replace the toothbrush as soon as the bristles spread out.

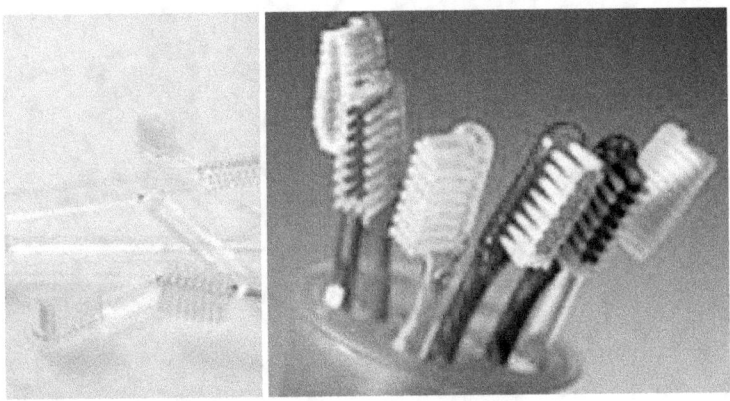

Although powered toothbrushes can generate more strokes than manual toothbrushes, it is best to use manual toothbrushes for children.

[65]

Contact Dr. Brazis at (916) 731-5151
Sign Up for To Tell The Tooth Newsletter at:
totellthetooth.com/sign-up

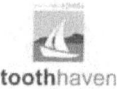
Mouthwash

Mouthwashes do not clean teeth. They only freshen your breath. Most mouthwashes contain alcohol and are therefore unsuitable for children.

===\\\===\\\===\\\===\\\===\\\===\\\===

Contact Dr. Brazis at (916) 731-5151
Sign Up for To Tell The Tooth Newsletter at:
totellthetooth.com/sign-up

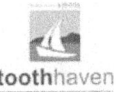

toothhaven

10. Dental Safety Tips for Your Child

Dental care is essential for your children. Yet, you should practice extreme safety techniques to make dental products safe for your children.

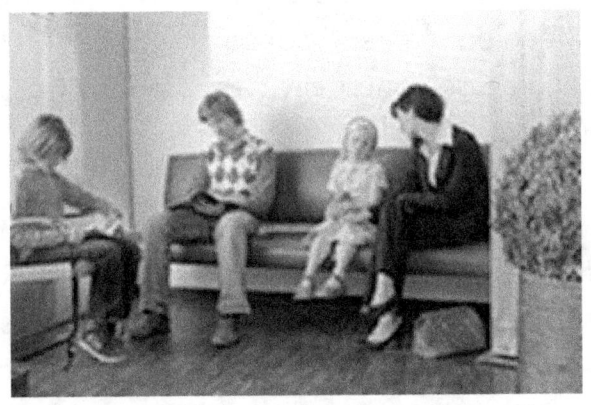

Dental Safety Tips

[67]

Contact Dr. Brazis at (916) 731-5151
Sign Up for To Tell The Tooth Newsletter at:
totellthetooth.com/sign-up

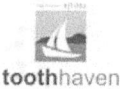
- Some of the toothpastes contain harsh abrasives that harm tooth enamel. Although these toothpastes claim to clean tooth stains, they also remove irreplaceable tooth enamel. Use non abrasive toothpastes.

- Keep mouthwashes out of reach of children. Most mouthwashes contain alcohol.

- Do not put your infant to sleep with a bottle of milk. Bacteria feed on sugars remaining in the mouth long after feeding and cause dental cavities. Use only water in bottles at bedtime.

- If using a pacifier for your infant, check nipples regularly. Brittle nipples can break and choke your child. Refrain from tying pacifier to your infant's neck. It could cause strangulation. Purchase and use pacifiers made of a single mold. Separate pieces fused together support chances of them coming away. Use pacifiers with holes in mouth guard area. This allows saliva to escape and prevents

Contact Dr. Brazis at (916) 731-5151
Sign Up for To Tell The Tooth Newsletter at:
totellthetooth.com/sign-up

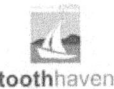
accumulation between infant's lips and pacifier. This prevents skin rashes.

- There have been some claims that mothers with gingivitis have higher risk of preterm deliveries. The mother's immune system can be affected thereby causing preterm birth. Although it is not yet fully substantiated and understood, it nevertheless makes good sense to treat gingivitis and minimize your body's infectious influence to the fetus. Hence, visit your dentist during your pregnancy to treat or prevent gingivitis and help your baby. It is well established that hormonal changes during pregnancy lead to an increase of gingivitis infections during this time.

===\\\===\\\===\\\===\\\===\\\===\\\===

[69]

Contact Dr. Brazis at (916) 731-5151
Sign Up for To Tell The Tooth Newsletter at:
totellthetooth.com/sign-up

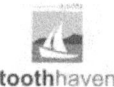
Part-V: Dental Care at the Dentist's Clinic

Contact Dr. Brazis at (916) 731-5151
Sign Up for To Tell The Tooth Newsletter at:
totellthetooth.com/sign-up

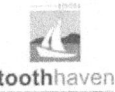

11. Types of Periodontal Diseases in Children

Periodontal diseases can occur in children as well as in adults. This disease manifests in children especially if your child also suffers from Down syndrome, Type I diabetes, or Papillon-Lefevre syndrome.

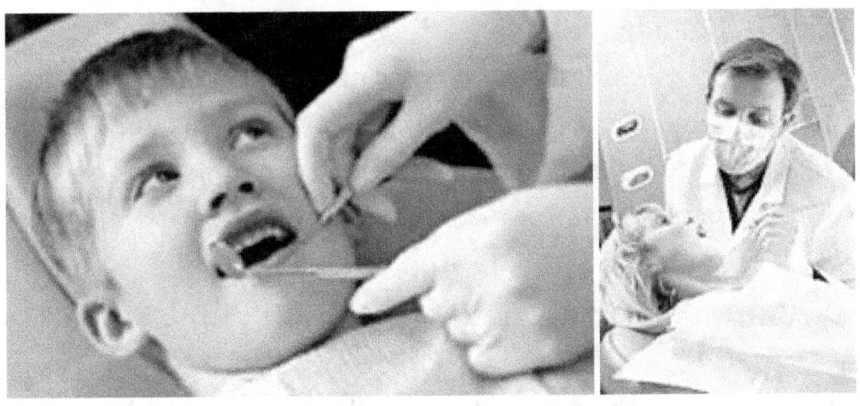

Different types of periodontal diseases include:

[71]

Contact Dr. Brazis at (916) 731-5151
Sign Up for To Tell The Tooth Newsletter at:
totellthetooth.com/sign-up

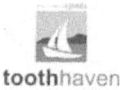

Chronic gingivitis: This causes swelling of gums and makes them turn red and bleed easily. Regular brushing, flossing and proper dental dental care can treat this disease.

Aggressive periodontitis: This affects incisors and 1st molars in teenagers. There is very little formation of dental plaque or calculus, so it can be detected only by regular professional examination. This disease affects alveolar bone.

Generalized aggressive periodontitis: This affects the entire mouth and does not restrict to any specific teeth or part of mouth. It causes inflammation of gums with heavy plaque accumulation and calculus. Over time, this causes loosening of teeth.

Symptoms of Periodontal Disease in Children

Constant bad breath despite regular brushing and flossing is a major symptom of periodontal disease. Hormonal changes

[72]

Contact Dr. Brazis at (916) 731-5151
Sign Up for To Tell The Tooth Newsletter at:
totellthetooth.com/sign-up

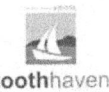

during puberty cause increased levels of estrogen and progesterone. This increases blood circulation to gums making them more sensitive to irritations and reactions. They turn more reddish and become tender. Practicing regular oral hygiene and good dental care can reduce such irritation considerably.

===\\\===\\\===\\\===\\\===\\\===\\\===

Contact Dr. Brazis at (916) 731-5151
Sign Up for To Tell The Tooth Newsletter at:
totellthetooth.com/sign-up

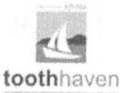

Your Children's Teeth: A Parent's Guide To Saving Money At The Dentist

12. What Should You Do if Your Child Has a Dental Problem?

Dental problems range in their degree of seriousness. The following tips can prove helpful:

- Dental problems in children could be hereditary. Regular brushing and flossing may not be enough to prevent serious cavities. Consult your dentist to correct the problem while your child is young. Heredity affects hardness of enamel, size, and shape of teeth and jaws. Problems may require dental restorations or orthodontic intervention.

- Children now do not always have to wear painful braces and metal wires to correct irregular teeth. There are various dental corrective appliances available in plastic. Dentists now advise dental corrections at a young age.

Contact Dr. Brazis at (916) 731-5151
Sign Up for To Tell The Tooth Newsletter at:
totellthetooth.com/sign-up

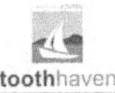

toothhaven

- It is now easy to fill dental cavities. Dentists have more choices for filling teeth. Materials for filling teeth include composite resins rather than the traditional silver-mercury alloy. Composite resins are bonded and hence, fillings do not have the tendency to pop out. Resins are available in a range of tooth colors.

- Dentists prefer using stainless steel and/or plastic crowns to cover teeth in case of malformation of baby teeth, fracture, or extensive decay. This maintains tooth form and position for optimal jaw development.

- If your child is into sports, encourage your child to wear mouth guards to help prevent injuries.

- **You should schedule regular meetings with your dentist to make your child comfortable with dental visits.** Practice good dental habits like regular brushing and flossing to prevent major dental problems. Also, limit the intake of sugary and sticky foods for your children, as these affect dental health immensely.

[75]

Contact Dr. Brazis at (916) 731-5151
Sign Up for To Tell The Tooth Newsletter at:
totellthetooth.com/sign-up

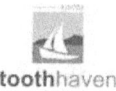

What Should You Do in Case of a Dental Emergency?

Dental emergencies can occur anytime and hence, being prepared beforehand is essential and helpful.

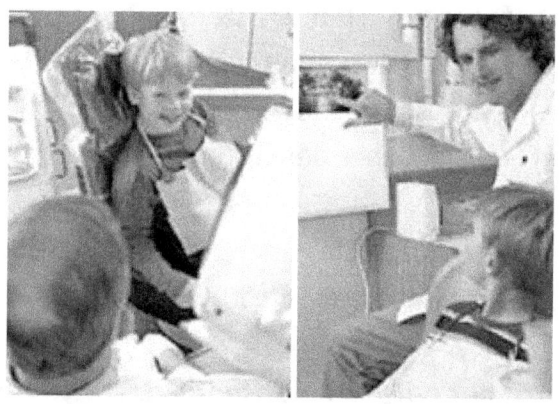

Taking Care of Dental Emergencies

Always <u>keep all contact numbers of your dentist</u> in a handy place so that it is easy to contact them in an emergency. Common dental emergencies in children include chipped

[76]

Contact Dr. Brazis at (916) 731-5151
Sign Up for To Tell The Tooth Newsletter at:
totellthetooth.com/sign-up

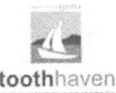
teeth due to accident and teeth knocked out or loosened due to trauma.

If a traumatic incident occurs, knocking your child's tooth out or just causing a loosening or mobility, contact dentist immediately within an hour, if possible. Dentist can re-implant tooth and save it. Until then, rinse tooth in water (distilled if possible) without touching tooth root. You can try to place tooth back into socket and secure it with a wet wrap. If this is not possible, preserve tooth in a cup of milk or saliva until you meet the dentist.

If your child feels pain due to a chipped tooth, it indicates possible injury or exposure of the tooth nerve. Meet with your dentist as soon as possible for evaluation for possible root canal treatment or similar measures to save tooth. Your dentist may treat the tooth temporarily and later fix a bonded restoration to make up for the chipped tooth. If there is no pain, set an appointment with your dentist and meet them at the earliest convenient time. The emergency is not as pressing, but future nerve damage cannot be ruled

Contact Dr. Brazis at (916) 731-5151
Sign Up for To Tell The Tooth Newsletter at:
totellthetooth.com/sign-up

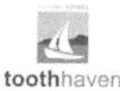

out until the dentist examines the injury even if there is no immediate pain.

If your child is into sports, ask him to use protective mouth guards. These plastic guards protect teeth as well as the lips, gums, and cheeks. Semi-formable mouth guards available at sports shops require boiling to give a perfect fit. Dentists also make mouth guards with molds that fit in snugly.

Dental emergencies can occur due to severe toothache arising from dental cavities, infections, food stuck between teeth, and broken fillings. Rinse your child's mouth every hour with warm water. Clean affected tooth area with toothbrush and floss thoroughly. Use toothpick to dislodge any food material stuck in between teeth. Use an ice pack on affected area to relieve pain. **Refrain from placing aspirin on child's gum, as it could cause aspirin burn.** If there is any swelling around eyes or cheeks, place ice pack. Ice packs should only be left in place for ten minutes at a

Contact Dr. Brazis at (916) 731-5151
Sign Up for To Tell The Tooth Newsletter at:
totellthetooth.com/sign-up

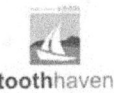

time, then removed for ten minutes. Then repeat the cycle. Take your child to a dentist immediately.

If you have small children, keep your home safe and free of furniture with sharp edges and corners as much as possible. Toddlers often suffer dental injuries while they are learning to stand. Children sometimes injure their teeth while ramming into water fountains while drinking water. Accidental bumping into each other could cause teeth injuries in children.

===\\\===\\\===\\\===\\\===\\\===\\\===

Contact Dr. Brazis at (916) 731-5151
Sign Up for To Tell The Tooth Newsletter at:
totellthetooth.com/sign-up

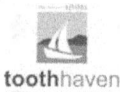

13. Taking Your Child to the Dentist

My advice to parents if they are comfortable with their own dentist is to bring their young children in with them for their cleaning visits. Many of my patients, who are new mothers, and sometimes even the fathers, bring their babies and young children along. The children tend to find being in a dental office quite natural and comfortable when it becomes their turn.

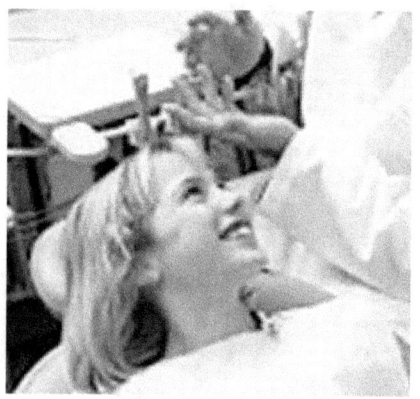

[80]

Contact Dr. Brazis at (916) 731-5151
Sign Up for To Tell The Tooth Newsletter at:
totellthetooth.com/sign-up

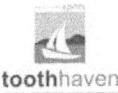

When the child is a little older, but still early enough that they have not developed any dental problems, the child can sit in the chair after their parents are done just to feel included. It is not forced, always voluntary and fun oriented, non-threatening. Later they can have their own appointment and by that time feel like they know the dentist and hygienist and are not afraid.

If there is a need for specialist treatment, dentists can refer to pediatric dentists, orthodontists, or oral surgeons for jaw realignment if your child has developmental jaw anomalies.

What Happens in a Dental Check-up?

Before visiting the dentist, prepare your child for the visit. Tell your child that the dentist will examine their teeth by "taking pictures" and then "counting their teeth." Using these words will help kids relate to what is going on much more than saying "x-rays" or "examining". Try to avoid

[81]

Contact Dr. Brazis at (916) 731-5151
Sign Up for To Tell The Tooth Newsletter at:
totellthetooth.com/sign-up

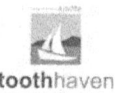
using words like "shot", "needle", "pain" and others like this when some kind of treatment is planned also.

At an initial visit, x-rays (*pictures*) may be taken, a visual examination (*tooth counting*), and possibly a cleaning (*tooth polishing*) can be done. Additionally, if the child is old enough, a topical fluoride treatment may be done, if the parent so chooses. Most dentists will be flexible with children's first visits to accommodate different children's ability to tolerate a new environment. The idea is to give your child a friendly, fun, non-threatening experience that they will look forward to repeating in the future.

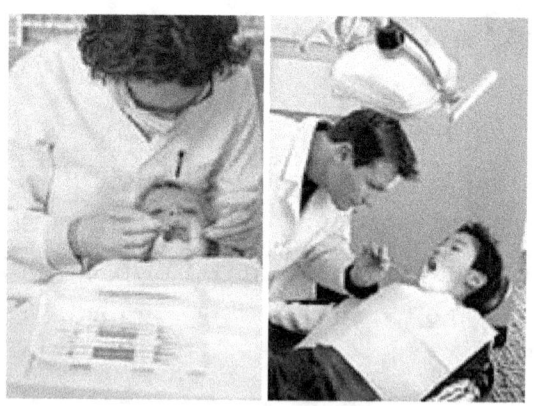

Contact Dr. Brazis at (916) 731-5151
Sign Up for To Tell The Tooth Newsletter at:
totellthetooth.com/sign-up

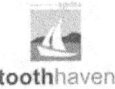

Encourage your child to draw pictures of mouth and teeth and allow your child to take these pictures to the dental office and talk to the dentist about them.

Before taking your child for a visit to the dentist, you could schedule a visit with your dentist and explain your fears and your child's first visit to the dentist. Dentists would take additional care to make your child's visit as simple and fearless as possible.

Never bribe your child to visit a dentist. Also, don't talk about a visit to the dentist as a punishment *(remember Sarah)*. Develop the habit of visiting a dentist right from the first birthday of your child.

Schedule biannual dentist visits when your dentist says they are ready. Your child becomes accustomed to visiting a dentist from a young age.

Contact Dr. Brazis at (916) 731-5151
Sign Up for To Tell The Tooth Newsletter at:
totellthetooth.com/sign-up

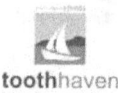

I hope reading this has been as valuable to you as writing it has been to me and that it contributes to your children's dental health. My goal is for everyone reading this book to come away with the realization that dental health and dentistry for children can be easy and fun and save a lot of money in dental visits over the years of your children's lives. I thank you for reading and wish you and your family good health and happy relationships.

===\\\===\\\===\\\===\\\===\\\===\\\===

A Special Offer For Sacramento Area Customers:

Bring this book into my office with you for your first appointment and your children will receive initial exam and x-rays for free.

If you are already a patient in my office, I will credit the cost of initial exam and x-rays of any of your children who are already patients in my practice or give free exam and x-rays to children not already in the practice.

[84]

Contact Dr. Brazis at (916) 731-5151
Sign Up for To Tell The Tooth Newsletter at:
totellthetooth.com/sign-up